# The Reactive Training Method

## 21 Secrets Revealed For Permanent and Easy Weight Loss

BY

ROBERT CLARKSON

ISBN: 978-1512168433
ISBN-13: 1512168432

# CONTENT

DEDICATION
ACKNOWLEDGMENT

# DEDICATION

For my beautiful daughter Kacey, she makes all the hard work
worthwhile☺

# ACKNOWLEDGMENTS

I would like to thank my friends and colleagues Maria & Kelly, who have both been on their own incredible journey but have always found the time to listen, help and support… Thanks x

# TESTIMONIALS:

**Lynsey Gillespie** "I spotted Reactive Training on Facebook when I was feeling very down and upset with how I looked and felt. It took a while for me to sign up as I was very nervous to start and I knew I had lots to do when it came to my fitness, nutrition and my self-confidence!! I was very scared on the first morning but the minute I arrived everything changed. I met Robert and the other ladies who were just as worried as me! Since then I have improved my eating, lost inches, lost lots of body fat and I have also made friends and feel much better about myself. In this last month I have achieved more than all the other years of slimming clubs put together. Robert and Maria are so nice and although they push you they also support you and every session is fun as well as hard work!! I had no idea I could do half the things I can now and have just signed up for another six months. It feels, right now, like the best thing I've ever done so thank you Robert and all the Team Reactive crew!!"

**Lorraine Buckley** "Thoroughly enjoyable experience. Love the atmosphere of class and other members involved are very encouraging and positive. Robert and Maria are nothing like other trainers I've experienced in the past, this is a whole new happier experience. You are never alone, if you're not sure about something all you have to do is ask your question on Facebook and you'll be helped out. The fitness and nutrition really do work hand in hand but it's just so much better when you're actually having fun doing it instead of going to the gym or weight loss classes."

**Rosemary Mackenzie** "Decided in November 2014 to try this and signed up for the 4 weeks trial which began on the 5th January - a New Year, a New Me! Slightly apprehensive on my first night, but Robert and Maria were so supportive - and everyone was there to improve their own wellbeing. From never having even seen a Kettlebell I was confidently swinging them at the end of the second week! The classes are never the same; circuits, boxing, kettlebells: even Yoga! The nutrition aspect of the trial worried me slightly, however it was a great boost to see everyone's photos and ideas on the Nutrition page. So - what did it do for me? I've now lost 8 pounds, and have a good reduction in not only my body fat but also my overall BMI. I've signed up for three months and am now confident in achieving my target - to be a fitter, leaner, not so creaky me throughout 2015 with vastly improved nutrition habits. Warning - attendance WILL result in a new wardrobe ;)

**Ann Mathieson** 'Nearly at the end of my four week trial and have enjoyed the whole experience. I came across it on Facebook and wondered if it was a scam till I checked out the reviews - now I'm adding my own! Have learned more about nutrition and have NEVER done so much exercise in my life. I am by nature pretty lazy and was trying to work out which classes I could miss and still qualify for the free trial, at the start. I attended 15 out of 16 classes and missed one only because I was held up at work. The classes have great variety and Maria and Robert make sure your technique is right and won't cause you injury. They encourage rather than push you. I lost weight, my body fat and BMI have dropped, my clothes feel looser and I can feel some fledgling muscle starting to grow and tone - my 'bingo wings' are shrinking too!

The classes are fun and supportive - I would recommend it to anyone who is ready to make a change in their overall fitness and health.

**Katie Naughton** "I stumbled upon Reactive Training's website in my search for personal training in Glasgow, and I was immediately impressed by it's positive and supportive feel. I decided to join, and am so happy I did. If you're like me and intimidated by the gym or choreographed classes, and are interested in working with a personal trainer, I highly recommend checking out the group training at Reactive. Robert and Maria keep it fun and varied, and even though you're in a group, you still get the personal trainer experience. It's definitely not easy, but the way I feel after only 2 weeks proves that it's worth it!

**Carol Harkins** "Support and encouragement is excellent, is more than a diet/exercise class it is an education and potentially a life change experience.

## Chapter 1: Why should I lose weight?

The first problem is the word WEIGHT because most people associate it with being a negative word, and automatically assume that being overweight is bad.

Being underweight can be just as damaging to your health as being overweight, but let me explain a little more.

At Reactive Training we like to use the words healthy or unhealthy as it takes into account more than just your physical weight on the scales.

Your weight is just a numerical representation of your relationship with gravity, it's not a representation of you as a person.

It can also be deceiving as it does not take into account lean muscle mass or fat mass.

Most people when they think about the numbers on the scales think of the weight as excess fat, which is not always the case.

We use various measurements and methods such as your weight and body fat percentage to determine if you are currently at risk in terms of your health.

Sticking to the BMI scale which uses your weight and height to determine your health, is a very good starting point for those who are currently inactive.

To keep things simple a BMI score over 25 is classed as unhealthy, the higher the score the higher the risk.

From now when we talk about being overweight, you can assume we mean unhealthy…

Everyone has different reasons for wanting to lose weight, some people even think they are happy being over or under weight…

Now I totally get that being comfortable in your own skin is one way to deal with your weight problems, but hopefully I can convince you of the benefits of getting and staying healthy and that it's not as difficult as it may seem.

Most people initially start their weight loss journey wishing simply to look better naked, there is nothing wrong with wanting to look a certain way, although at Reactive we encourage you to look a little further than just vanity…

Sure looking great naked is a great reason for starting but here is some equally as important benefits to shedding those pounds ;)

Firstly your health, being overweight or obese greatly increases your risk of:

Heart Disease, Stroke, Type 2 Diabetes, High Blood Pressure, Osteoarthritis, Cancer, Back Pain, Depression and lots of other minor ailments and conditions.

Your life expectancy is significantly reduced… (YES YOU WILL DIE SOONER)

Not only that but the quality of your life is restricted and impaired.

Losing weight and getting healthy will help you live a longer fuller life…

Now let's look at some of the other benefits to losing weight and becoming healthy:

Increased energy and productivity in all aspects of your life, suddenly playing with the kids and grandkids is now FUN. (no more feeling like you can't keep up)

Improved confidence from looking and FEELING your best, no more hiding under baggy clothes (you CAN wear that dress).

Increased sex drive, combined with all that extra attention your partner won't be able to keep their hands off you.

Improved stress and ability to deal with any situation, bad days at the office become a thing of the past.

Increase in alertness, memory and learning capacity meaning you no longer forget those important tasks, become more productive and everything now becomes easier.

You become the role model you want to be for your children, good habits rub off and all of a sudden the kids and grandkids are interested in YOUR new hobby, they want to exercise and eat just like YOU.

Increased relaxation and recovery, say goodbye to sleepless nights and insomnia.

Exercise releases endorphins and serotonin, which is known as the happy hormone, it makes you feel good about yourself and banishes those negative thoughts.

Improved self-esteem, by taking back control you start to feel good about yourself again and the skills you learn are transferable to all aspects of your life.

You get to meet awesome likeminded people just like you, because you can never have enough good friends ;)

In short you become the person you always knew you could be, happy, content and back in control.

## Chapter 2: What do you recommend to someone who feels too unfit or overwhelmed to even start?

Almost every single person who has ever joined any of our programmes has not felt ready and feels overwhelmed; these are exactly the type of people we are trying to help.

It's normal to feel this way; it's a huge misconception that you have to be fit in order to join any sort of fitness regime.

We are fooled into to seeing skinny supermodels and celebrities in magazines and social media that we delude ourselves this is the norm.

The truth is that fit and healthy is the minority; we live in a society where obesity is on the rise with over 60% of the UK classed as obese.

Just like it's wrong to stereotype someone who is overweight as being lazy, you shouldn't assume that every training programme is extreme and beyond your capabilities.

Great trainers take into account exactly where you're starting from, and I have never met anyone yet who is unable to change and improve their health.

Our training programmes are designed to challenge every person no matter their ability, every single one of us is unique and as such we all require a personal approach to becoming healthy.

One of the reasons I started Reactive Training was due to so many people feeling unfit and overwhelmed.

I wanted to create an environment that was unlike your mainstream gyms and classes.

An environment that offers all the benefits of 1 to 1 personal training within a group setting.

I have created a community that is supportive, understanding and above all welcoming to women just like YOU.

No matter your starting point YOU can still take action and make changes.

Reactive Training offers additional support when needed to help with your confidence in attending our training camps.

I can assure you that your fears of being the worst in the class or the biggest will be put at ease within seconds of meeting the team.

You will quickly realise that everyone is there to help and support, every single journey no matter how near or far starts with that first step…

The hardest part is taking that first step, the training is actually the fun part and you will be amazed how much you will actually enjoy training with our group.

We have members who hated exercise in the past and built up such a negative view of exercise that it held them back, now they can't believe that they actually look forward to coming and hate the thought of missing any sessions.

In today's world with so many promises, which fail to deliver, it's totally understandable to feel overwhelmed and out your comfort zone, but I ask you not to let it hold you back…

Think about the consequences of not taking that first step?

Think about your reasons for wanting to become healthy?

## Chapter 3: I feel like there is nothing I can do about my weight, what do you recommend?

There is no secret formula or magic exercise but every single person needs just one thing in order to lose weight and become healthy, without it I am afraid it's not going to happen.

"If you want things in your life to change, you have to change things in your life"

You have to be willing to change your lifestyle, if you're not willing and still continue to live an unhealthy lifestyle while hoping to become healthy, then sorry it's not going to happen.

Making changes doesn't mean you have to be boring, survive on chicken and broccoli everyday and never drink alcohol again.

When you have been overweight for some time you forget what being healthy feels like, you start to accept that this is the norm.

No person is meant to be overweight and unhealthy, to make ourselves feel better we tell ourselves stories and excuses that it's ok, that it's just the way you are.

Being overweight does not mean you're a bad person or any lesser than someone else.

It does make you unhealthy and greatly affects your health, wellbeing and how you feel.

The good news is that everyone has the ability to change.

You might have tried several methods before that have failed, you might feel like no matter what you do it just never seems to work.

Simply put you have just been trying the WRONG things for you.

With the right support and education you can change it around.

Remember trying to ride a bike for the first time?

It felt like you would never do it, like it was an impossible task.

But with a little perseverance, guidance and support you finally said goodbye to those training wheels ;)

Many people go wrong and have a bad experience because they try to do too much; they go along to a mainstream class and try to keep up with the regulars who have been going for years.

You end up overreaching, pushing too far while every muscle in your body aches and your walking kind of funny for the next few days…

You have tried some extreme new diet, that you hate but

decide to give it a go because it worked for so and so…

You just end up binging at the end of the week because your starving and feeling deprived.

Our training although in a group, is personal and bespoke to you. Everyone works at their own level and the programming is tailored to ensure that you are always making progress.

Now combine it with specific nutrition just for YOU, no shakes, potions or food you can't stomach.

We educate you on what foods are best to keep you feeling great throughout the day, while helping to give you energy to support your training and shed that unwanted body fat.

There is no more diets, just sensible flexible nutrition so that you can have your cake and eat it ;)

All of our training and nutrition works because it is repeatable; it's not something that you do for 6 weeks while hating every minute.

It's a genuine blueprint on how to live your new healthy life in order to feel great, at times you might even think it's too easy…

## Chapter 4: I'm afraid that I'll fail and maybe even feel worse if I start a weight loss program, what can I do?

Do you want to be healthy everyday or just for a few weeks?

What about feeling better?

If you are always looking for that quick fix is it any wonder you perceive weight loss as a SUCCESS / FAIL scenario.

You're kind of setting yourself up to FAIL before you even start.

Like everything mentioned already we try to get you to change your mindset and look at things differently.

Fear of failure is worse than failure itself, and fear is a very powerful emotion.

Failure is not the problem it's the fear, so instead of being scared to fail think about being terrified of remaining unhealthy, dying young and never being the person you know you can be.

Don't let the negative thoughts of not being good enough or strong enough hold you back from starting…

I promise that no matter what happens you will feel better, be brave and believe in yourself.

Failure is actually part of the programme, not in terms of weight loss or health but life.

It's what you do after the failure that counts.

You will fail at some point, it's through this failure that we learn and grow. There is no magic formula or secret supplement for health. The key is consistent practice and education of healthy living, everyone has occasional blips it's what makes us human.

If you are constantly seeking perfection and 100% adherence is it any wonder when you have a night off you feel worse?

Its ok to make mistakes and have the occasional blip, in fact sometimes we even encourage you to relax and enjoy yourself.

It's not ok to throw the towel in and give up just because you have one bad day, the support and guidance helps you through those tricky times to get back on track.

A bad day is not the end of your journey, it's just a minor detour we just recalculate another route and pick up from where we left.

You will learn skills that you will have for life, skills like riding a bike you never forget, that you can come back and use to help you achieve your goals.

If we consistently chase health and feeling good then weight loss will happen naturally without seeming like it's consuming your life.

When you start to think of your health as a journey as opposed to a destination you move away from the quick fix mindset.

Too many people want instant results, but just like gaining weight never happened over night neither will becoming healthy.

There is no such thing as a quick fix, if there was a ready-made solution to cure obesity then it would already be available.

If you come into our programme with the right mindset, ready and willing to make changes while being realistic and patient you won't need to be afraid.

That's why we have a stringent selection process, because in order for us to truly help, you have to be willing and ready to look at lifelong changes.

## Chapter 5: How can I start my own weight loss if I don't have the time or energy to do it?

Do you know what the number one excuse for not starting a weight loss programme is?

"I don't have the time"

Do you know about the self-fulfilling prophecy?

"A false definition of the situation evoking a new behaviour which makes the originally false conception come true"

Sometimes we perceive that we have no time, we even find other things to do to fill our time, fulfilling the misconception that we have no time.

How many hours of TV do you watch each week?

How many hours do you spend on Facebook each week?

How many hours do you spend feeling shit about yourself each week?

A recent study has shown that more than 50% of an average waking day is spent using media (texting, talking, typing, gaming, listening or watching) that's more hours than we spend sleeping each day.

The good news is there is normally always a way to steal some time or use it more productively, to promote health.

For example we use activity trackers with our members, we monitor how active you are throughout the day just by monitoring your steps.

Everyone should do a minimum of 10,000 steps everyday, and it's amazing how creative you become to hit your target.

So parking the car a little further away each day, taking the stairs, standing at your desk, extra comfort breaks, pacing while on the phone are just some of the tactics used to find time to be active.

No matter how little time you think you have, you still have to eat. By implementing our healthy choices you are already taking action and working on your weight loss.

It's very rare that someone actually has no time to start; if they genuinely do think so then my suggestion is they need to find balance and make time for their health.

As for not having enough energy, this is a direct consequence of your lifestyle choices, and is easily fixed by starting a programme to improve your health.

Being inactive promotes feeling tired and lethargic as opposed to being active, by adding in more activity your body will respond by giving you more energy.

Eating quick processed foods also causes you to crash and burn, you get a quick release of energy from the sugary foods but because you're so inactive your body releases insulin to store the energy which causes you to feel tired and lifeless.

Our nutrition programme is designed to give you energy at the right time of day, avoiding those crashes. You will feel like you have a new lease of life, and the food you eat will nourish your body and promote health.

By embarking on this journey you will not only have more energy but more time, the benefits will spill over into all areas of your life and the only thing you will regret is that you never started sooner.

## Chapter 6: I want to start my journey to weight loss but I'm afraid that I will be injured or sore, what do you think?

Being injured and sore from exercise sucks PERIOD.

The soreness you get from exercising is what we call DOMS (delayed onset muscle soreness) and is a muscular pain caused by micro trauma in your muscles.

Now unfortunately a lot of trainers think that the sorer you are from training then the better the workout.

Now this is just plain crazy, and rest assured dumb and not the intention of a well-planned bespoke training programme.

Initially some form of discomfort is to be expected, especially if you have been very inactive for some while.

But walking like a cowboy for days and struggling to sit on the toilet are not signs of a good training programme.

After a few weeks as your body starts to get used to being active then the DOMS are very rare, and tend to happen when doing only new types of exercise (that your body is not used to).

Most of the members just follow our recommendations to keep moving and the discomfort goes away, however we do have a couple of strategies for those really worried.

Magnesium is a supplement we recommend which can be used as a spray, which your rub in to the muscles or as bath salts that you soak the muscles in.

Both are really good for speeding up recovery while minimising soreness, and if you have been really inactive and are worried a really good inexpensive option to use.

In terms of injury our focus is always on technique and the quality of the movement, injuries are rare and generally we find that new members who have previous niggles and minor injuries tend to quickly see them disappear.

We believe that movement is the best form of exercise and have seen members go from relying on a walking stick to unaided within 4 weeks.

We also work closely with a local Physio and provide a monthly clinic to work on mobility and any issues outwith our scope of practice.

Injuries should not deter you from being healthy and can always be worked around, we recently helped one of the members through a broken foot injury.

Although unable to use her lower body, we adapted her programme to focus on the movements she could do and adjusted her nutrition to support her new activity levels while injured.

During her injury she continued to lose fat and gain health each week.

Overall a good programme will help you move better, prevent injuries occurring, help to heal current injuries and should not leave you in any sort of lasting pain or muscle soreness.

## Chapter 7: Do you recommend fast weight loss?

It all depends on what you mean by fast?

We certainly would not recommend anything dangerous or promote a quick fix.

You may have heard or even tried some of these weight loss shakes, potions or diets?

Sure some of them will get you results but at what cost?

Are you robbing Peter to pay Paul, and in a few months' time you put it all back on because the methods and products are unsustainable?

We tackle fat loss on many fronts, looking at your overall lifestyle including nutrition, activity and recovery.

Sometimes you may get results by focusing on just one aspect but to really improve health you have to include all 3.

The reason the quick fix potions never work long-term is that they are not sustainable, are you really going to skip meals and drink shakes for the rest of your life?

The reason you are unhealthy and overweight is your lifestyle, the only true way to sustain changes and feel good is to change your lifestyle.

Every single person is different and some can make changes quicker than others, some have more fat to lose than others.

If a person embraces the change, becomes more active, eats healthy and gets adequate recovery then generally 1-2lbs per week is a great target, some who have more to lose such as extremely obese can be as much as 3-4lbs per week.

Weight loss is not always so linear and as previously explained; weight does not take into account lean body mass (muscle).

Ideally we wish to reduce our fat mass while increasing our lean body mass, it is not uncommon to lose 1-2lbs of body fat while gaining the same in muscle.

This at first can seem very disheartening especially if your sole focus is on the numbers shown on the scales, because it would appear that you have not made any progress.

The truth is you have actually made huge progress by increasing your muscle mass, while decreasing your excess body fat. It's your excess body fat that causes you to be unhealthy, the more lean muscle and less body fat you have the less jiggly you will be.

You will start to notice the difference in your shape and how you look, they say it takes about 4 weeks for you to notice, 8 weeks for your friends and family to notice and 12 weeks for the rest of the world to notice.

You should notice a difference in how you feel within the first few weeks, again trying to get away from what the numbers say on the scales focus on how you feel and if you're feeling good 90% of the time the fat loss will take care of itself.

## Chapter 8: Do the fat burning pills and protein shakes work?

There are many supplements that claim to promote fat loss and with so many out there it's easy to get confused about what's good and what's bad.

First let me quantify what I mean by good and bad, just because something works doesn't necessarily mean it's good.

Smoking for example, has been proven to help with weight loss but I am sure you don't need me to tell you about the health implications.

A good supplement is something that will support your health and work alongside your nutrition and exercise, to improve your results.

Let me start with the fat burning pills first, generally they are a combination of stimulants with a high caffeine dose that yes can provide a fat burning effect…

The problem is that they also place a huge amount of stress on your body's adrenal system, which has been shown to cause long term damage and in some cases death.

Personally they are just not worth taking the risk, especially if you are already out of shape and not in good health.

Now lets talk about protein, which tends to get a bad reputation due to being associated with the bodybuilding world and meal replacement rubbish.

If you think about protein supplements, you tend to picture some muscle bound guy necking back his shake after the gym or Herbalife / Juiceplus.

Let me quickly touch on Herbalife / Juiceplus as these are what we call meal replacement shakes, and although they contain protein are totally different and shouldn't be thought of in the same way.

Herbalife and Juiceplus use genetically modified soya protein, it's very cheap and massed produced, and it is also filled with lots of preservatives, chemicals and loads of other rubbish you can't even pronounce. They are not a good choice of supplement and should be avoided at all costs.

Good protein supplements come in many forms the most popular being whey protein which comes from milk, you can also get other good forms such as casein, beef, pea, hemp, rice etc.

They all come in powder form, and are usually mixed with water to make a shake.

Why would you want to supplement with protein powder you might ask?

Simply put, most women struggle to eat enough protein to support fat loss and exercise.

Of all the weight loss studies carried out on both successful low carb and low fat diets the consistent element was a high protein content.

What is a high protein?

The recommended daily allowance RDA set by the government is 0.8 grams of protein per kg of body weight each day.

Don't get me started on the government guidelines for nutrition, like everything else they are always way off the mark.

The International Society Of Sports Nutrition ISSN position stand takes a different view:

Protein intakes of 1.4 – 2.0 grams per kg of body weight per day for physically active individuals are not only safe, but may improve training results.

When part of a balanced, nutrient-dense diet, protein intakes at this level are not detrimental to kidney function or bone metabolism in healthy, active persons.

Supplementing protein is a practical way of ensuring adequate and quality protein intake (hold that thought).

Additionally a very recent study by Jose Antonio (2014) goes a little further and actually shows that even with a very high protein diet, subjects had no adverse effects or weight gain.

The group consumed 4.4g/kg/day of protein which is 5.5

times the recommended daily allowance, and still never increased their body fat, even though their total calories were higher.

You can check out the study here:
http://www.jissn.com/content/11/1/19

Additional benefits of eating more protein is that it will keep you fuller for longer, stop you eating excess calories from carbs and fats, maximise your recovery and improve your results.

So basically even if you overshoot and overeat on your protein requirements it won't have any adverse effects… (note it's not a free pass to eat your bodyweight in Nandos)

Here's the thing, most women are not even hitting anywhere near their requirement, which means they are filling up on other sources (carbs and fats) which generally have a higher calorie content.

A good target for our members would be to aim for 2g/kg/day so for Maria weighing in at 70kg (11 stone) her target would be 140g per day. (aiming for the higher target gives you some wriggle room and ensures you're at least hitting 1.4g/kg/day)

But what exactly does 140g of protein look like?

(note 100g of chicken does not equal 100g of protein)

Canned Tuna = 20g (84kcal)

2 x Chicken Breast = 40g (182kcal)

3 Eggs = 20g (225kcal)

Ground Beef = 20g (196kcal)

Small Greek Yoghurt = 20g (111kcal)

2 x Small Tesco Brazil Nuts = 17.5g (826kcal) or 1 x Whey Protein Shake = 20g (83kcal)

Now this is a lot of food to eat just make sure your hitting your daily protein requirements, most women would definitely struggle, never mind trying to fit in your healthy carbs and fat requirements.

This is where protein supplementation comes into play, in the form of a protein shake, it allows you to still hit your daily requirements and actually keeps your calories in check.

Caution in order to get less than 20 grams from a few handfuls of brazil nuts you would have to consume 826 calories (this is more calories than all of the other foods combined).

You can get the same amount of protein from a nice chocolate (or whatever flavour you like) whey shake for less than 100 calories!!!

Yep so you're basically getting more bang for your buck from the protein shake while keeping your calories in check (remember that weight loss is determined by your total overall calories).

At Reactive Training we try to stay away from the whole calorie counting and focus on sensible flexible nutrition, it doesn't seem sensible to me to eat half your daily allowance from a handful of nuts ☺

Protein shakes are used to supplement your nutrition plan and should not be confused with Herbalife / Juiceplus meal replacement shakes.

So having protein at every meal with a few protein shakes ensures you're hitting your requirements while keeping your calories in check to support weight loss.

(tuna, turkey, chicken breast, white fish and seafood like scallops or shrimps) are the best sources of protein for weight loss as they provide the "leanest" sources of protein with the fewest carbs and calories.

I already know that quite a few of our members are intolerant to milk and dairy which rules out whey protein, not to worry there are lots of great quality alternatives such as rice, hemp, pea and even beef protein powder (it doesn't taste of beef).

There are lots of places to buy; most supermarkets are often very overinflated in price.

Take away points:

Are you eating enough protein, to support your goals?

Are you eating protein at every meal?

Is it worth looking at supplementation?

## Chapter 9: What is the best exercise for weight loss?

Have you heard of the super inverted upside down squat?

It's the best exercise you're not doing to get amazing results…

Unfortunately it does not exist, there is no single BEST exercise, and instead we need a combination of basic fundamental movements and nutrition to provide best results.

Master the basic movements and STRENGTHEN and you have a simple formula to give you the best form of exercise women can do to get amazing results.

The Kettlebell is such a great tool as it can be used to provide resistance to the basic movements such as push, pull, squat, hinge and carry and can be used in so many other ways.

Many people still think that cardio training is the key to fat loss; did you know that too much cardio could actually be detrimental to your results?

Surely you must have seen some women instructors who teach 20+ classes a week and still seem to be chunky?

They call this "Chunky Fat Aerobic Syndrome" no joke it's a real condition.

With too much cardio type classes your body quickly adapts and you become really efficient at what you do.

So basically you become great at doing classes, but because you're so efficient your body has no need to dip into your fat stores for energy and you can even start to store more fat.

For fat loss we want the body to become inefficient, meaning that you become a fat burning machine. Strength training places such a demand on the body that you are burning fat for days after each session.

Other benefits of Strength training are you become stronger, your bones and muscles are no longer weak, this transfers to everyday life and tasks become easier.

As you burn fat and increase muscle tone, your shape will change and you start to look athletic. Think of Jess Ennis as opposed to a body builder, you wont get huge you will tone, lift and not sag giving a more youthful appearance.

With strength training it also increases your cardiovascular fitness (your heart and lungs ability to repeat a given task) so you get more bang for your buck.

Unfortunately it doesn't work the other way, so any cardiovascular training will not make you stronger.

Group aerobic classes such as Body Pump, Body Attack, Insanity, Step etc. are predominately aerobic in nature.

Even though you are lifting weights in some of these classes it is not sufficient to produce the correct training effect.

They also promote poor quality movement, because it's all about how much and how many reps you can do without emphasising on the quality of the movement.

If you repeatedly train poor movement with half reps, poor technique then the only thing you will improve is that you will be able to do more poor quality movement or if your unlucky you might get injured.

Proper STRENGTH training that focuses on improving your movement quality while making you stronger is the key to success.

Women initially are scared at the thought of lifting weights and working on strength, a good coach will not only make it less intimidating but will make it fun.

Other misconceptions about STRENGTH training are that it's best suited to athletes and younger women. This is absolute rubbish, STRENGTH is the only quality that you can continue to improve as you age and anyone can start at any time.

Strength training focuses on quality as opposed to quantity, the workouts are designed with lots of rest and at times you even think it's a bit easy. Don't be fooled by the initial difference, it's because of this simplicity it becomes repeatable.

When your workouts become repeatable they also become sustainable long term, so to answer your question what's the best exercise?

The exercise you continue to do week after week ;)

## Chapter 10: What tips for losing weight can you share?

Stop focusing on weight loss for a start, sometimes you can't see the forest for the trees.

If you put all your focus into feeling good each day then the fat loss will take care of itself.

The best tips for long lasting health and feeling good each day is to make long lasting changes.

You have to work at all aspects of your health, nutrition, movement & recovery each and every day.

If you only focus on one area and neglect the others then you will stagnate and lose focus, you have to be genuinely ready to make changes.

This doesn't mean that your life is over and you cant go out or have fun anymore, it just means that you have to choose your battles and 80% of the time follow your new healthy lifestyle.

It leaves you some room 20% to relax and enjoy life, holidays, birthday parties, nights out you can still have fun and know that it won't affect your long term results or health.

Look at the bigger picture and focus on making small progress consistently rather than huge progress for a few weeks, giving up and constantly starting again.

Nutrition should be about eating to feel good, you're no longer on a diet it's just how you eat to feel your best.

Movement is about exercise that makes you stronger and improves your quality of life, like being able to squat down pain free, walk up the stairs without being out of breath, roll around on the floor with the kids without feeling like you can't get back up.

Recovery is about getting good quality rest and relaxation, sleeping well so you feel rested and ready to tackle anything put in front of you.

Patience is needed as it takes time to change the bad habits of a lifetime, sometimes when you try to make too many changes at once you can start to feel overwhelmed.

Instead just focus on making small improvements each week and don't beat yourself up if you have to take a few steps back.

A good example would be with your nutrition, if you know you need to cut out some bad habits like too much fizzy juice and sweets then start off gradually.

Try to reduce the fizzy juice first and replace with water, it may take a few weeks and you might still sneak the odd can or glass which is ok.

Once you feel you have it under control then it's time to try something else, like cutting out sweets or cooking new meals.

Apply the same principle to movement and recovery; small actions that you can repeat everyday are more beneficial in the long run.

It also helps to add accountability in, as if you try to do it yourself it's easy to skip or miss out when you have a bad day.

By getting yourself a great coach, not only will they keep you accountable they can speed up your progress and get you there faster and support you on your journey.

## Chapter 11: Is there a meal plan for weight loss that works better than others?

Every single person is different, and we all have a different need that's why some diets work for some people and not for others.

At the heart of every single successful diet for weight loss there is a calorie deficit.

Which means that your body requires more calories than you are consuming, so in order to make up the shortfall your body dips into your fat stores for energy.

It works the other way too, so when you consume more calories than you need your body stores this as excess fat.

Now it's not always as simple as calories in verses calories out, as like I have mentioned before exercise and recovery has a huge role to play also.

If you are very inactive then your body will require fewer calories, if your active and exercising then you require more.

Every single weight loss plan has some sort of deficit built in, be it Weight Watchers, Slimming World, Atkins, Zone Diet, 5:2 Diet etc.

The reason they work is that over a period of time you eat less than your body needs, the problem is that although some of these plans can work they are not the best choice or specific to you feeling your best every day.

The reason they don't work for some people is they are not compatible or sustainable long term, some are too extreme and just impossible to keep up.

Technically you could lose weight eating chocolate cake every day, just as long as you don't over eat…

But how would you feel?

Think about food in terms of how it makes us feel, do you feel tired, sluggish, bloated, foggy or depressed?

Or do you have energy, mental clarity, focus, strength, happiness, and wellbeing?

All foods have an effect on how you feel, sometimes we just have not connected the dots yet, next time you have a meal think about how you feel within one hour of finishing and for the rest of the day.

Rather than a diet, I like to promote a lifestyle of eating that supports you to feel good while reducing your body fat to a healthy level.

We focus on single ingredient foods, home cooking and anti-inflammatory foods that support recovery and prevent illness.

No calorie counting or points, no traffic lights, just simple eating to feel your best every single day.

We post regular recipes on our blog, we have a Reactive cookbook and the food and meals are delicious.

Once you get used to cooking and making your own dishes, it is really simple and quick to maintain.

There is nothing that is banned or disallowed within moderation, so you still have that 20% to relax and enjoy some treats and we even teach you how and when to have treats without it impacting on your health and results.

## Chapter 12: Is there a difference between weight loss and fat loss?

Yes, your weight takes into account everything in your body, muscle, bones, organs not just your fat stores.

Excess weight is not necessary the problem it is excess fat that causes us to be unhealthy while increasing your body size to look unflattering, it's the fat that makes you jiggle.

As previously discussed muscle is a lot denser than fat so a smaller amount of muscle in terms of volume can actually weigh more than fat.

We use both BMI and body fat percentage to determine initial health risks for our members.

Generally a BMI of 25 or less is considered healthy, we would also look for a body fat percentage of less than 30% initially as a good indication we are heading in the right direction.

It is possible to have a BMI over 25 with a body fat percentage under 30% this would be an indication that the individual has a higher percentage of muscle mass.

This is mostly found in people with experience of training especially lifting weights, for most people who are overweight with no experience of training they would normally have a high BMI and high body fat over 30%.

Our first initial target with 90% of our members is to get within the healthy range of both BMI and body fat %.

From there it gives us a good starting point, in terms of fat loss and our ideal goal for health would be to increase lean muscle while losing fat.

This will drastically change your appearance, your body will tone up, loose areas will tighten, your muscles will lift to give a more feminine sexy shape, you will start to see definition and jiggling will be a thing of the past.

We want to preserve your lean muscle, and you do this by incorporating strength training into your programme. If you are not performing resistance training and eating enough protein you run the risk of losing muscle mass alongside fat.

This can be detrimental to how you wish to look, as can leave your skin looking saggy; you can even become what is known as skinny fat. Skinny fat is when you start to lose muscle mass while still maintaining stubborn jiggly fat especially around the belly and buttock areas. This can also lead to health problems.

Yes we want to focus on fat loss, but this will also show on the scales depending on your starting point especially if you have a lot of excess fat to lose.

That's why it's important to not just focus on weight loss only, but also use a combination of measurements to monitor your progress.

Using a combination of measurements, such as your

weight, body fat percentage and your hips and waist circumference will allow us to have a much more accurate view of progress.

## Chapter 13: What are three factors you think will help someone to be successful in their weight loss?

We live in the age of instant information; if you want to know anything all you have to do is "search it up", as my daughter would say. Nutrition, Movement & Recovery is certainly important but you already knew that. To really be successful the most important 3 factors are accountability, education and taking action on all 3 pillars of health.

The 3 pillars of health (weight loss) are nutrition, movement and recovery they are interlinked like Borromean Rings. The 3 rings together are inseparable, but remove any one ring and the other 2 will fall apart. There is no hierarchy and all 3 should be given equal attention in order to fully benefit your health and wellbeing.

The first step is taking action, deciding to change and learn how to be the best you can possibly be, a good coach will keep you accountable in all 3 areas while educating you and giving you lifelong skills.

Nutrition is about eating to feel good, single ingredient whole foods that nourish your body and soul to give you energy, vitality and keep you feeling your best. We all know that we shouldn't really eat sweets, takeaways and drink fizzy juice, but sometimes it doesn't stop us.

Movement is about being active, going back to fundamental basics and getting stronger in those movements. In modern society the majority of people have lost the ability to perform basic fundamental human movements such as squatting, pushing, pulling, hinging and carrying. If you look at any young children move they are graceful and can do these movements with ease while supporting their own body weight. Our modern lifestyle forces us to become inactive and we lose these basic movements. For our health it's important we reclaim them and get back to mastering the basics, too many want to run before they can walk. It's not all about doing the new fitness craze with complicated movements, faster and harder. Keep it simple master the basics, then get stronger doing those movements, keep it simple and don't over complicate things.

Sleep / Recovery in order to lose weight you have to recover properly, not enough sleep causes a stress response which forces your body in to storage, and can prevent fat loss. Without adequate recovery your body will not repair and heal, your efforts to get stronger and leaner will be wasted. Sometimes it can really be as simple as fixing your sleep patterns to break out of a weight loss plateau.

A great coach will provide you with all the factors needed to be successful; they will challenge you to learn, keep you accountable and encourage you to keep taking action.

## Chapter 14: For someone who experiences their weight going up and down, what advice can you give?

It is normal for your body weight to fluctuate by a few pounds here and there; of course when you are healthy this is not a problem. The problem arises when we have extremes, such as yo-yo dieting which produces great short-term weight loss followed by a large increase in weight most often more than what you started with. This is why DIETS don't work, because they are not designed to follow long term, so you get good results and you think you have reached your goal. You have no long-term solution so end up going back to eating the way you did previously that caused weight gain.

Sustained health and wellbeing comes from a lifestyle change, it's a way to live for the rest of your life and shouldn't feel in any way restrictive. There has to be flexibility built in for those unexpected life events and to allow you to relax and enjoy yourself in moderation. At Reactive Training we encourage the 80/20 principle, so that 80% of the time you are following a very healthy nutritious lifestyle, with the 20% reserved for you to relax and enjoy the not so healthy foods in moderation.

When you take away the restrictive constraints of a "DIET" you empower people to make their own choices, they know that they can have a drink of alcohol if they wish or a dessert but are sensible and it's part of their new lifestyle.

This approach also removes the mental barrier associated with "DIETS" because in the past when a traditional diet becomes so difficult to maintain and you eventually crack you beat yourself up for days that "You're Weak" or "You Have Failed" when in actual fact your normal like everyone else.

Deprivation is a short-term fix, but we seek long-term health and results. We have to shift our mindset and look at the long game, once you accept that to get healthy and stay healthy all you have to do is BE healthy, everything becomes so much easier.

I love the quote "We Are What We Repeatedly Do" if you binge drink every weekend, eat takeaways and occasionally go on a diet then I'm afraid you will always be on the roller coaster of yo-yo dieting.

Ask yourself this question…

Over the last 12 months how have I repeatedly lived my life?

Now ask yourself this question…

Do I want to feel the same for the remainder of my life?

If you want to feel, look and be the best version of you then realise that it takes consistent repeatable effort over the long haul.

Don't get this confused with the difficulty you have experienced with dieting, feeling deprived, tired, crabbit, hungry and miserable. This is not the way to live your life 80% of the time, jeezo it's not even worth it for a few weeks if you ask me.

Instead when you learn how to eat to feel good, you will get lean, feel less bloated, your skin and hair will shine, your ailments will disappear, you will have sustained energy and moods throughout the day and be well on your way to reaching your goals.

## Chapter 15: What are the keys to permanent weight loss?

Firstly education, with so many new fad diets and information it is easy to get confused. Weight loss is a billion dollar industry and so many businesses are competing for your hard earned cash. Unfortunately the majority of companies don't really care about the long-term success because it's not good business sense. Most of the big sliming clubs want you to fail as it keeps you coming back for more, lining their pockets. Education is needed in many areas; firstly nutrition and how to adopt a healthy balanced lifestyle that will allow you to FEEL your best. This is not as easy as just prescribing which foods to eat, it's an individual process and what works for one person is not necessarily the best for others. Combined with nutrition education is the psychology of weight loss, changing people's perceptions which they have lived with all their life. Working on habits and dealing with expectations and failures along the journey is also important.

If only it was as simple as education, we also need support and guidance, which is best not only from a coach but a group environment. Being part of a bigger team where everyone has similar struggles helps to spur each other on. It also helps to motivate and make the whole experience more fun, (yes losing weight can be fun). It also allows you to see that other people just like you can achieve and reach their goal, this builds confidence and reassures you that

YOU can despite what you may tell yourself.

Now we need to apply this model of education, support and guidance to not just nutrition but movement, recovery and lifestyle as combined they become so much more powerful, this may seem like a lot of hard work but that's where a good coach comes in…

A great coach makes the process, fun, easy and enjoyable see next question.

## Chapter 16: Do you recommend us having a personal trainer?

I don't really like the term personal trainer, as there are just so many stereotypes associated with it.

What's the first thing that pops to mind when you think about a personal trainer?

1. Ex-Military Sergeant Major, Sir YES Sir...

The fact I used to actually be in the military, I hate this. Yep I joined straight from school as a fresh faced 17 year old and served 6 long years.

But I couldn't be further away from the type of military instructor you imagine, it's not about screaming and shouting in your face while kicking dirt in your eyes :)

2. Gym Fanatic...

I am not someone who lives in the gym, lives off of chicken and broccoli while posting selfies and videos of my latest lifts. Sure I train, but you would hardly even know ;)

3. Mr Motivator…

Loud music and shouting while dancing around like the energiser bunny is not me either, anyone can scream and shout plus I can't dance :)


4. Cross Fitter...

Writing an almost impossible workout on a white board then trivialising it with a niche female name: Agatha, Beryl, Eugenie, or some other rubbish.

5. Body Builder...

Wearing vest tops even in winter, looking in the mirror every 2 seconds while flexing my huge guns and don't forget the protein shake I constantly carry around.

Nope none of them are me...

Instead I like to think of myself as a coach...

At Reactive we don't do all the other stuff, we coach people to reach their potential.

Coaching comes in many forms; it might be nutrition based, strength based, movement or even life coaching.

It is certainly not any of the above, and sometimes this has caused confusion.

You see most people have a predetermined expectation of exercise and what they should do to reach their goals...

Almost everyone we have ever worked with has got us totally wrong; this can be both good and bad depending on how much you are willing to change your mindset.

Let me explain why it's sometimes a problem ;)

You think all you have to do is train more and eat less?

You have the mindset that it's all about training harder, working till you feel sick and walking funny for days after (the sorer the better).

When they come to Reactive we strip it back and focus on mastering the technique of the basic movements (which BTW everyone struggles with).

You don't always get sweaty; you are not always out of breath so surely it can't be good?

A great coach doesn't care how many you can do; they care about how you do it.

Anyone can work you hard, make you feel sick ITS NOT COACHING.

Initially it can be tough having to go back to basics, the ego doesn't like it...

But if you try to build a temple on shitty foundations it's only a matter of time before it all comes crashing down.

Should you get a coach?

Absolutely YES

Sure you could figure it out yourself, everything you need to know is on the World Wide Web...

But how long will it take YOU?

A good coach will keep you accountable, and fast track you to stardom light-years before you will get there yourself.

Do you really want to struggle, continue to feel like shit and keep on starting over?

Investing in a coach will be the best investment YOU ever make, and the education and results will outlast those new shoes and dress ;)

## Chapter 17: How can I choose the best personal trainer for me?

You have to do some research, initially you can search on google or Facebook or ask friends and family for any recommendation.

Check out the coach / trainer website, Facebook page and look for testimonials, the testimonials should come from women similar to you. No point in going to a trainer who predominately works with young male athletes and has no experience of working with women. Contact one of their customers to ask some questions about their experience and journey, and to gauge if the coach would be a good fit for you.

Do they offer?

Body fat and weight measurement?

Nutritional coaching?

Lifestyle coaching?

1 to 1 coaching?

Group coaching?

Ask about the type of training and experience, do they do exercise classes?

Or is it specific group training?

Once you have narrowed it down then give them a call and ask to meet up for a chat about potentially joining up.

A good coach will be informative and offer you the opportunity to ask questions, they should even have an option for you to come along and try what they do.

Be wary of cheapest in town, like anything else you get what you pay for and when it comes to your health you don't wanting be shopping in the whoopsie aisle.

Generally you will get a good feeling and know the right trainer for you after you do your research and meetings.

## Chapter 18: Is having a personal trainer expensive?

Not having a personal trainer (coach) is expensive…

What's the cost for you to not make changes and carry on the way you are?

I love this quote by the Dalai Lama when asked what surprised him most about humanity… "Man surprised me most about humanity. Because he sacrifices his health in order to make money. Then he sacrifices money to recuperate his health."

When you actually sit down and work out how much money you spend on stuff that is moving you away from your goals versus money you spend on moving closer to your goals you will be surprised.

The problem with most people is that they want to look and feel their best but continue to live an unhealthy lifestyle…

When you lead a healthy lifestyle and make some sacrifices to help you reach your goal, and start to shift from a cost mindset to an investment mindset then finding a great coach will be worth every penny.

Like any profession you have various levels of service, good and bad coaches, it's important not to shop on price as you run the risk of getting a personal trainer that does not have the experience or skills to help you reach your goal in the shortest and most efficient way.

What's better?

A personal trainer at £25/week over 24 weeks or a personal trainer at £50/week over 12 weeks?

Firstly having a cost mindset can in the long run end up costing you more, take for example all the fad diets, shakes, pills and potions that seem like a bargain at the time…

How did they work out for you?

When you add up the cost in both finances and time you have already spent trying to reach your goal, the realisation can be frightening.

A Skoda and a Ferrari can both get you to your destination, but which will get you there quicker? Provide you with the best experience and really leave you with a journey you will never forget?

You can also find most information on the Internet these days, and try to figure everything out yourself, but again how long is it going to take you?

The most expensive commodity you have is your time, the less time you spend struggling and in pain the better.

Personally I want the fast pass to health, I prefer to get the expert help and support to allow me to reach my goal far quicker than I could do myself.

Not only will it save me money in the long run, but it will give me more time being healthy, feeling my best and allowing me to spend that time with those I love as the best possible version of me.

## Chapter 19: How can I choose the best weight loss program for me?

Now with so many different weight loss programmes and products out there it becomes difficult to make a decision, so you have to ask yourself what do you really want?

If it's just a quick fix for an upcoming holiday or wedding then a lifestyle approach is not going to work.

Especially if you're not ready to make changes and just want to lose weight, a recent study actually showed that most women would chop off their arm to lose weight…

Pretty drastic considering they are not ready to commit or willing to make changes that will lead to the same outcome.

My philosophy around weight loss is always to get healthy first, let me ask you this question…

Do you know anyone who is healthy, who is overweight?

My approach is to chase health, get stronger and feel fantastic and the byproduct is fat loss.

So of course I am going to recommend that the best weight loss programme is a lifestyle approach, because not only will you become healthy you will look and feel your best and have the skills to continue to do so for the rest of your life.

Do you just want to look good for the holiday or for the rest of your life?

The problem with my approach is that it takes time, it takes investment to actually learn the skills necessary to live a healthy lifestyle.

We live in a world where we expect everything yesterday, and too many people are just not willing to make lifestyle changes.

They want a quick fix, they want the magic pill…

But…

It doesn't last, the effects are temporary just like Cinderella at the ball everything will eventually come back and sometimes more, and then how do you feel?

If you really really want to get off the roller coaster of YoYo weight loss programmes then you have to invest in your future, be in it for the long haul and learn the skills to keep you feeling fantastic all year round.

A great coach will accelerate this process, make the journey fun, enjoyable and challenging enough for you to learn without throwing in the towel.

It should feel right, not like a diet or something you hate…

You should be making progress and learning, taking responsibility rather than following a plan, and for me this is the key to success.

What's the best programme for you?

That all depends on what you really really really want ;)

## Chapter 20: What are the factors that stops one from losing weight or even getting started on a program to lose weight?

There are so many reasons that prevent someone from losing weight; I'll try my best to cover the main reasons.

At the very basic level weight gain can be down to inactivity, overeating or a combination of both.

Inactivity can be down to many reasons such as sedentary job and lifestyle, when you become sedentary your calorie needs is less.

If you continue to eat above those needs the result is weight gain.

It doesn't happen overnight, it's a very slow gradual process and just kind of creeps up on you, but before you know it you are not the size you used to be.

In order to reverse the process it requires changing these bad habits, which may have been going on for years.

Unfortunately it's not just as simple as eat less move more, there are so many more factors that need to be addressed.

It's not easy, and most people have made the mistake from being inactive to trying to be very active.

This causes a negative experience with exercise, as we become sore due to how much we are de-conditioned and the thought of more exercise is terrifying.

Changing eating habits can also be scary especially if you are of the mindset that you are being deprived, no one likes to be told what they can and cannot do so when traditional diets exclude your favourite foods you rebel.

Everyone is at different stages and for some have tried all the diets and quick fixes possible, which not only leaves them feeling like shit but they don't believe that anything will work. They have convinced themselves that they are just FAT and that they will always be this way, what's the point in trying if it's not going to work? They have had their fingers burnt so many times that they have lost all hope, not just in the process but also in themselves.

Others really want to start but are terrified of the environment; they are used to seeing the Biggest Loser on TV or have experienced a traditional gym environment and are not comfortable. They worry they will be the fattest and everyone will judge them, that they won't be able to do what's required, will be shouted at by the scary instructor and eventually fail and feel worse.

Some don't want to give up their lifestyle, eating convenient meals, takeaways; drinking through the week and weekends has become the norm. They want to feel better but fail to associate this lifestyle is what is causing the pain and suffering. They think it's ok to drink a bottle of wine after work because they have earned it, and why should they have to give it up? Deep down they know they are self-sabotaging but are just not ready to let go.

Some are not ready to invest both financially or time into the process. They think nothing of spending money or finding time on stuff that takes them further away from their goal, they just haven't prioritised their health at this moment in time. Everyone has different financial circumstances but there is always an option available to everyone if you are really ready...

For example: If you simply have no means to hire a coach you could volunteer at a local college or university to work with the student coaches as a case study, most would jump at the chance to have clients to work with while learning their profession.

Finally the main reason which kind of covers all the rest is that we tell ourselves some sort of story about what it will be like, what the outcome will be and attach a negative feeling around the whole process.

The truth is that it's actually nothing like what you think, the difficulties and troubles you perceive are just in your head, the fear is created by your mind and is paralysing.

Every single member we have ever worked with actually enjoys the process, weight loss and becoming healthy does not have to be your worst nightmare.

It should be an experience that although challenging is enjoyable, educational and rewarding.

## Chapter 21: Can you tell me about your approach and Reactive Training when it comes to losing weight and being healthy?

At Reactive Training our approach is slightly different from the traditional weight loss programmes.

We use a lifestyle transformation system, that will address all factors relating to your health.

When you chase health, not only will you lose weight you will gain so much more.

Our approach is also coaching based, it's about teaching the importance of leading a healthy lifestyle and how to maintain it.

"We are what we repeatedly do"

So By Being Healthy... We Are Healthy

One of the hardest tasks is changing the mindset and perception of weight loss; almost every member is so focused on the numbers shown on the scales they struggle to see the bigger picture.

We firstly address inactivity, and use Fitbit (a fancy pedometer) to measure how active or inactive you are each day. The minimum activity levels we should all maintain is 10,000 steps each day. As previously discussed the lack of activity plays a big part in weight gain, with the Fitbit we are able to monitor each member every day and have a very clear understanding of their current activity.

The good thing about this is that anyone can use it, it's just simply walking or moving around but it is this lack of movement, which leads to problems. It's especially good for members who feel they are unable to start any exercise programme, and is a gentle introduction to moving more.

The Fitbit activity monitor also monitors your sleep patterns, adequate quality sleep is really important for your health and it's amazing the improvements just by making some little tweaks to your nighttime routine.

We then look at nutrition and educate on how to eat to FEEL good, we don't believe in diets or counting calories (unless you have performance goals like an athlete). We initially use an elimination protocol over 4 weeks, eliminating inflammatory foods that are known to cause issues such as bloating, IBS, tiredness, skin problems and many other minor ailments. The initial 4 weeks is a little restrictive but is designed to cut out the foods causing most damage to your health, it also allows you to gauge how you feel when not consuming certain foods. We educate during this process about the different types of macro-nutrients protein, carbohydrates and fats and their benefits.

Rather than the traditional diet model, where certain foods are limited or banned we explain and educate you on the importance of eating to feel your best. Nothing is off the menu but overconsumption of certain foods will have consequences, it's important to rebuild a healthy relationship with food as opposed to thinking good and bad. It's also important to install responsibility for you to realise that you are in control of your nutritional choices and that the occasional blip is not only part of the learning process but also a normal part of life.

With education you learn to not beat yourself up over food, feel more in control and confident that you can easily implement your new learned strategies to help keep you feeling your best, while supporting your training and fat loss.

Alongside daily movement and nutrition we implement a more detailed movement based training programme. This takes the form of small group sessions based in our Glasgow studio. We work with women on their basic human movements and then use various modalities to strengthen and improve these movements.

Our philosophy is movement based, the reason people become de-conditioned and overweight is their lack of movement. This approach goes against many other opinions within the fitness industry, which traditionally take the more is better approach. Meaning that so many classes, bootcamps etc focus on the intensity and totally neglect the quality and type of movement.

Very often it's more about getting you out of breath, sweaty and sore… You might even hear sayings like "No

Pain - No Gain" or "Pain Is Weakness Leaving The Body" this approach especially when you already have poor movement quality leads to you feeling out your depth, in pain and waiting for an injury to happen.

Instead we meet you where you are, and every single session is designed in order to challenge your movement quality. It can be very different from anything you have experienced especially if you are used to exercising in the traditional manner. Sometimes it requires you to leave your ego at the door, because when you strip back your technique it really shows up your lack of movement and strength. When you have been used to doing lots of poor quality movements and feeling like you are making progress it can be a shock to the system having to start as a beginner again. That's why we are very particular in who we work with, because anyone who wishes to join has to be coachable. They have to be willing to address their weaknesses and strive to move better. Our sessions are very technical and require patience and re learning of basic movements. We use tools like the Kettlebell to strengthen your basic movements and get your stronger and leaner. This makes up the foundations of our movement system, then we add in additional activities such as boxing and yoga. These work in synergy and fit perfectly with our philosophy of movement and strength, while also being really fun.

To discover more about 'The Reactive Training Method' and take your first step your health and freedom go to:

www.reactivetraining.co.uk

# ABOUT THE AUTHOR

Robert's journey with exercise and health began with active military service, and has spanned professional and community based sport, private health care and academia. His studies include postgraduate work and extensive vocational qualifications under some of the world's foremost leaders in health and fitness. He lives in Glasgow and continues to Lecture part time while running Reactive Training.